Sugar Detox

The Ultimate Beginner's Diet Guide Recipes

Solution To Sugar Detox Your Body & Quickly

Beat the Sugar Cravings Addiction Naturally

By *Simone Jacobs*

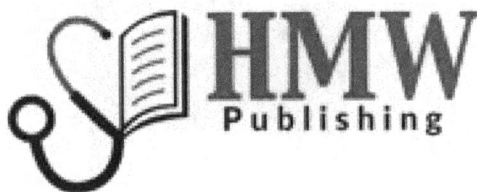

I0134901

HMW Publishing

For more great books visit:

HMWPublishing.com

Download another book for Free

I want to thank you for purchasing this book and offer you another book (just as long and valuable as this book), "Health & Fitness Mistakes You Don't Know You're Making", completely free.

Visit the link below to signup and receive it:

www.hmwpublishing.com/gift

In this book, I will break down the most common health & fitness mistakes, you are probably committing right now, and I will reveal how you can easily get in the best shape of your life!

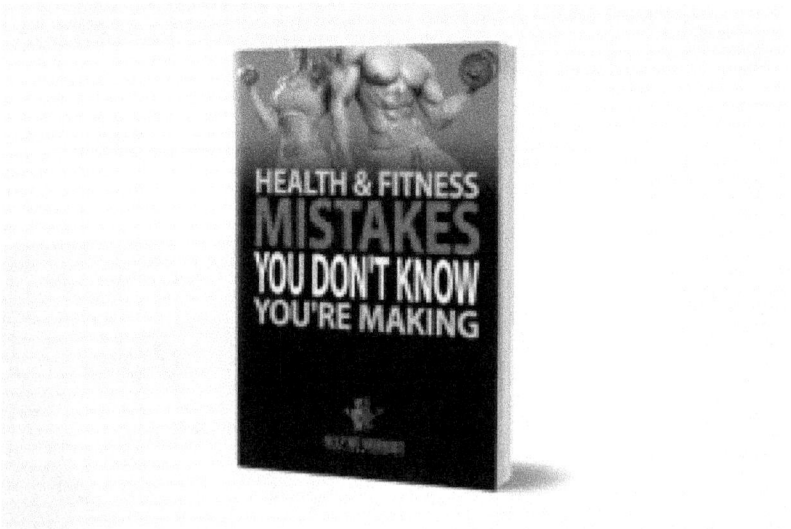

In addition to this valuable gift, you will also have an opportunity to get our new books for free, enter giveaways, and receive other valuable emails from me. Again, visit the link to sign up:

www.hmwpublishing.com/gift

Table Of Contents

INTRODUCTION

This book contains proven steps and strategies on how you can successfully overcome your sugar addiction. This Sugar Detox guide will help you discover how you can still eat delicious meals and become healthier.

Moreover, you'll learn the advantages of kicking junk, sugary and processed foods out of your life. Likewise, will also explain and reveal how to deal with the symptoms of sugar detox. Lastly, this book will also provide you with delicious meal plans, action plan, and Sugar Detox-friendly recipes to help you get started right away!

Also, before you get started, I recommend you **joining our email newsletter** to receive updates on any upcoming new book releases or promotions. You can sign-up for free, and as a bonus, you will receive a free gift. Our *"Health & Fitness Mistakes You Don't Know You're Making"* book! This book has been written to demystify, expose the top do's and don'ts and to finally equip you with the information you need to get in the best shape of your life. Due to the overwhelming amount of mis-information and lies told by magazines and self-proclaimed "gurus", it's becoming harder and harder to get reliable information to get in shape. As opposed to having to go through dozens of biased, unreliable and un-trustworthy sources to get your health & fitness information. Everything you need to help you has been broken down in this book for you to easily follow and to immediately get results to achieve your desired fitness goals in the shortest amount of time.

Once again, to join our free email newsletter and to receive a free copy of this valuable book, please visit the link and signup now: **www.hmwpublishing.com/gift**

CHAPTER 1: SUGAR – THE ROOT OF ALL HEALTH EVIL

Oh, sugar! How do I love thee? Let me count the ways. Studies reveal that the average American consumes about 22.7 teaspoons of sugar daily. Even without adding sugar to your food, you are eating processed foods that are packed with sugar to enhance the flavor and texture of the food and to act as a preservative to extend its shelf life.

To give you a picture, here are the most common food you consume every day and their sugar content:

Food	Size	Amount of sugar (1 teaspoon = 4.2 grams)
Ketchup	3 tablespoons	1.77 teaspoons
Oreo cookies	3 cookies	2.49 teaspoons
Low-fat fruit yogurt	8 ounces	6.16 teaspoons
Cola	12 ounces	7.93 teaspoons

Lucky charms	1 cup	2.55 teaspoons
Wheat bread	2 slices	0.66 teaspoons
Pork and beef bologna	4 slices	1.18 teaspoons

The natural foods you eat also contain natural sugar. For example, 27 grams of corn, 1, 135 cups of rice, 454 eggs, and 7 red apples contain 22.7 teaspoons of sugar.

If you are not mindful of what you eat, you can easily consume excessive amounts of sugar than what your body needs. **According to the American Heart Association (AHA), men need 9 teaspoons or 37.5 grams of sugar and women need 6 teaspoons or 25 grams of sugar daily.**

Our bodies need sugar or glucose to function. To understand the importance of sugar, let's take a quick look at what sugar is and in what forms we need to make it for the best benefits, specifically glucose and fructose.

What is Sugar?

Sugar is a pure form of carbohydrate that comes in many ways.

The Six (6) Kinds of Sugar

- Glucose – occurs naturally in plant juices and fruits. This pure sugar can be carried in the blood. It is the other half of the sucrose or table sugar, paired with fructose.

- Fructose - occurs naturally in cane sugar, fruits, honey, and root vegetables. It is the other half of sucrose, paired with glucose.

- Galactose – combines with glucose to form lactose. This is also known as milk sugar, and it makes up 5 percent of cow's milk.

- Sucrose – or commonly known as table sugar. This sugar naturally occurs in sugar cane and beets.

- Maltose - made up of two joined glucose molecules.

- High fructose corn syrup – this sugar is chemically

very similar to sucrose. However, half of the glucose is converted to fructose.

All carbohydrates, once consumed, are converted into glucose during digestion, which is the sugar that our body needs.

The problem is we consume food with too added sugar. We add table sugar in almost every food we eat – from coffee, tea, baked goods, and more. Table sugar is composed of 50 percent glucose and 50 percent fructose.

Glucose, as mentioned before, is metabolized throughout the body – the glucose is absorbed from the intestines into the bloodstream and then distributed to all the cells of the body. Glucose is vital to the proper functioning of the brain since it is the primary source of fuel of the billions of neural nerve cells in the brain. Neurons can't store glucose themselves, so they need a constant supply from the bloodstream.

Blame It on Fructose

Fructose is processed mainly by the liver and is turned into fat, which can build up and enter the bloodstream. Moreover, the market is also flooded with products – from soda to soup, with high fructose corn syrup. High fructose corn syrup is cheaper and sweeter than sucrose made from sugar cane and beets. What's the difference? Not enough to fuss about since they both contain fructose and everyone can benefit from eating less, if not eliminating it, from their diet.

When you consume too much fructose, it causes various health risks, including type 2 diabetes, insulin resistance, hypertension, and obesity. In fact, nephrologist Richard Johnson from the University of Colorado Denver, states that when you trace the path of the illness back to its primary cause, you will find your way again to sugar, fructose in particular.

Sugar Addiction: A Not So Sweet Love Story

If an extra slice of cake or chocolate has tempted you, then you know exactly how addictive sweets are and how difficult it is to cut back. To put it just, sugar in our bloodstream stimulates the same pleasure centers in the brain that responds to cocaine and heroin.

Sugar is not all bad for us. In fact, our body needs sugar. Johnson theorized that our ancestors evolved to become an efficient processor of fructose for survival, storing even the smallest amounts it as fat during times when food is abundant for use during the scarce seasons. Thus, today, we have a craving for fruit sugar.

For some people, sugar can end up in a full-blown addiction, the same way someone is addicted to abuse drugs like cannabis, amphetamine, and nicotine. There is no difference. The only dissimilarity is that sugar is legal and is not a controlled substance. In fact, people who are addicted to alcohol and drugs claim that craving for junk and sweet foods is similar. The worst part, sugar is not a regulated product. Often, we consume sugary foods without knowing the risks that it poses to our health.

How Does Sugar Destroy Us? Let Us Count the Ways.

Sugar is a bad habit, and it's a bad habit that's hard to break. Most of the time, we don't realize that overeating sweets and junk food are not a problem. To give you an idea just how bad sugar is for your health, here are some of their long-term effects.

Bad for Your Teeth

Added sugar, high fructose corn syrup, and sucrose contain calories without any essential nutrients. Hence, they are called empty calories – they contain no essential fats, vitamins, minerals, or protein – just pure energy.

When you get 10 to 20 percent or more of your calories from sugar, this can cause nutrient deficiency and health problems.

Sugar is also bad for the teeth because it is a source of digestible energy for the harmful bacteria in the mouth.

Cause Liver Problems

As mentioned earlier, sugar is broken down into two simple

sugars, fructose, and glucose. We need glucose in our body while there is no physiological need for fructose. Moreover, fructose can only be metabolized in the liver, where it is transformed into glycogen and stored in the liver when not used.

It is not a problem if you only eat small amounts of fructose from fruits and you are physically active. However, if you overeat fructose-rich food, you will overload your liver, forcing it to turn the fructose into fat. When you repeatedly eat a significant amount of sugar, it can lead to a non-alcoholic fatty liver and cause various health problems.

Keep in mind that it is almost impossible to overeat fructose from eating fruits since they contain very little fructose. The problem starts when you consume foods with too much sugar additives.

Cause Insulin Resistance and Diabetes

Insulin is a hormone that is vital to various bodily functions. It helps blood sugar or glucose to enter the cells from the bloodstream. It also tells the cells when to begin burning glucose instead of fat.

When you have high levels of glucose, the body works overtime to produce insulin, flooding the cells with the hormone. Thus, the cells become resistant to it. When you are insulin resistant, it leads to various diseases, including obesity, metabolic syndrome, cardiovascular disease, and especially type II diabetes.

Cause Cancer

Insulin does not only regulate the glucose levels in the body. It also controls the growth and multiplication of cells, which is the characteristic of cancer.

Many scientists believe that if you consume too much sugar, the constant high levels of insulin in the body can cause cancer.

Excessive Weight Gain and Obesity

Not only is fructose metabolized differently from glucose. Studies also show that fructose does not have the same satiety as glucose. People who drank fructose-sweetened beverage felt hungrier and less satiated than people who drank glucose-sweetened drink. Furthermore, the fructose does not lower ghrelin, a hunger hormone, as efficiently as glucose can.

Over time, because fructose isn't as filling, you will feel the need to increase your caloric intake, eating more food, which, in turn, causes weight gain.

Many studies reveal that sugar is the main cause childhood obesity. Kids who drink sugar-sweetened beverages are 60 percent more at risk of obesity. If you want to lose weight, the most important thing you can do is to reduce sugar consumption.

Raises Cholesterol Level

For a long time, people blamed saturated fat for heart disease, which is the number one cause of death in the world. Recent studies reveal that saturated fat is not to blame. Evidence suggests that SUGAR and not fat, is the leading cause of heart disease, due to the harmful effects of metabolizing fructose.

Studies reveal that high amounts of fructose raise the triglycerides, dense, small low-density lipoprotein and oxidized LDL, increase the levels of glucose in the blood, insulin levels, and abdominal obesity in as short as 10 weeks.

Consequently, various observational studies reveal a healthy relationship between high sugar consumption and the risk of heart disease.

Aside from the chronic diseases, most of the people who are addicted to sugar experience the following symptoms:

- Heart rate changes

- Mood changes

- Vision changes

- Seizures and convulsions

- Diarrhea

- Poor equilibrium/dizziness

- Weakness and fatigue

- Rash/hives

- Joint pain

- Memory loss

- Headaches and migraines

- Vomiting and nausea

- Insomnia/sleep problems

- Weight-loss problems

With all the health problems that can be traced back to our love for sweet foods, there is a need to detoxify from sugar. Our bodies have evolved to get by with just the smallest amount of fructose. The problem is that our world is flooded with high fructose corn syrup and sucrose. It can be challenging to break up with sugar, but it is an effort that we need to do for our overall health.

CHAPTER 2: WHY YOU NEED TO END YOUR LOVE AFFAIR WITH SUGAR

Now that you understand how too much sugar and sugar addiction can be detrimental to your health, it is time for detoxification and rehabilitation. It will take considerable effort and willpower to reset your body from a state of chaos. However, rebooting your system will benefit you in the long run.

The Benefits of Sugar Detoxification

Regulate Insulin Production

Mentioned earlier, too much sugar increases the production of insulin, which can often cause insulin resistance and lead to diabetes. Too much fructose also turns into stored fat. When you detoxify, the output of insulin in your body normalizes, which reduces the storage of fat in the belly and food cravings.

Improve the Insulin Sensitivity

When the body has high levels of insulin all the time, the cells become resistant to it. Thus, the body is unable to regulate blood sugar levels efficiently. Rebooting your system allows the body to adjust the production of insulin, which improves blood sugar regulation, helping you lose weight and improve your health.

Normalizes Cortisol Production

Cortisol is a hormone produced by the adrenal glands and the levels of the cortisol in the body rise and fall during different times during the whole day. It is at its highest level in the morning to help you get ready and move at the start the day, and it is at its lowest at night to help you wind down for a good night's rest. When your body has too much blood sugar, it weakens the adrenal glands, which affects cortisol production, a hormone that also helps regulate the blood sugar on a metabolic level.

When the adrenal glands are tired, it is unable to produce the right amount of cortisol that you need in a day. Hence, you will feel sluggish and low in energy. Instinctively, you will want to reach for a quick fix and most of the time. You will munch on a carbohydrate snack, coke, sugary food, or coffee. This is only a temporary solution, one that leads to a spike in blood sugar and insulin production, which later ends up with your blood sugar crashing and ultimately, weakening your adrenal glands even more. The result is a continuous low cortisol production, which is evident in the morning when you wake up feeling tired and unrested even after a night's sleep.

When you detoxify, the system resets, helping your adrenal glands recover and enable it to supply your body with the right amounts of cortisol at different times of the day.

Lowers the Production of Ghrelin, the Hunger Hormone

When you consume sugary food, your body increases its production of insulin so that the sugar can be converted and used by the cells of your body. It also increases the levels of leptin, a hormone that regulates fat storage and appetite, which decreases the production of ghrelin, controlling your food intake. The idea is that when you eat, your body automatically works to let you know that you should feel less hungry.

The problem occurs when you consume too much fructose. The cycle that should tell you that you are full does not happen. You already know that the body uses glucose. Glucose also suppresses the production of ghrelin and stimulates the production of leptin, which both works to suppress the appetite.

Fructose, on the other hand, not only affects the regulation of ghrelin, but it also interferes with the brain's communication with leptin, which leads to overeating. This is why fructose leads to excessive weight gain, insulin resistance, metabolic syndrome, and increased belly fat, as well as the long list of chronic diseases.

When you limit your fructose to healthy levels, it regulates and lowers the production of the hunger hormone ghrelin.

Cures and Prevent Leptin Resistance

Research reveals that when you consume fructose, you generate more fat in your liver compared to other types of sugar. Moreover, fructose blocks the body's ability to burn fat.

When you eat fewer calories, but you eat large amounts of fructose or your diet is high in sugar it will still cause a fatty liver, insulin resistance, and leptin resistance.

You have learned earlier that when you eat sugar the leptin levels of rising and signal your body that it is full so that you will stop eating. However, when you are leptin resistant, your body no longer responds to leptin. You end up eating more because you don't feel full or satiated. Hence, sugar detoxification will significantly benefit you.

Improves the Effects of Peptide YY or PPY

Peptide YY is a hormone released in the intestines and colon that controls appetite. When the sugar level in your body is unstable of high, it impairs the effects of PYY in appetite suppression.

Naturally Increases the Levels of Dopamine

Sugary and junk food changes the brain's chemistry, making you want more and more of them, even when you are full.

Dr. Robert H. Lustig, pediatric endocrinologist, and Dr. Elissa S. Epel, a psychologist, explain that when you consume large amounts of sugar, your brain releases massive amounts of dopamine, the hormone responsible for making you feel good. When there is a surge of dopamine, it causes the dopamine receptors to down-regulate.Meaning, there are now fewer receptors for them, so the next time you eat sugary and junk foods, their "feel-good" effect is blunted, thus, you need to eat more of them to get the same feeling of reward.

Sugar detoxification resets the reward pathways of the brain, allowing you to feel pleasure from eating real food.

Resets Tastes Buds

According to research at the Monell Chemical Senses Center, which was published in the American Journal of Clinical Nutrition, avoiding or eliminating sugar for a period will reboot your taste buds. When you consume low amounts of sugar for a couple of months, even foods with little sugar will taste sweet. This means that when you detoxify, you will be able to enjoy delicious treats more, you will be quickly satisfied with a smaller amount, and you will be less likely to overeat.

Reduce Inflammation

If you can recall your biology lesson about inflammation, you will remember that our bodies depend on temporary swelling to help fight infections and injuries – the inflammation cleans cellular debris, kill pathogens, and create protection to help to heal. Inflammation of a wound is a symptom that indicates the body has it is doing its job, the swelling, redness, slight tenderness, and warm feeling is the body's defense at work.

However, when the inflammatory response is turned on all the time? When you experience chronic inflammation, the immune system attacks normal cells by mistake, and the process that normally helps the body heals causes destruction.

Dave Grotto, RD, a spokesperson for the American Dietetic Association says the sugar cause inflammatory disease. When the body is unable to regulate the sugar and insulin levels in the body, a hidden inflammation in the body can cause chronic infections. When the blood sugar is high, the body generates more free radicals that damage the cells of the body, stimulating a response from the immune system, which causes inflammation that you cannot see.

Eliminating sugar, processed foods, and ordinary food sensitives, together with consuming foods that help fight off inflammation, reduce your risk of developing chronic diseases.

Boosts Detoxification

As mentioned in the previous benefit, too much sugar in the body increases free radicals. When you detoxify, you not only reduce the damage to your cells caused by free radicals, you also help your body get rid of other toxins that make you fat.

The benefits you get from detoxifying from sugar, as well as processed food, will help your body heal. When you avoid sugar, you will not only lose weight, but you will also benefit from the long-term health improvements.

Food You Need to Avoid

That is the question. To get the full benefit of sugar detoxification, you will not only need to avoid sugar. You will also need to avoid other types of food.

Sugar

By this point, you probably know why you need to cut back on sugar. However, it can be a scary change, especially if you have a sweet tooth. Don't worry; you won't go crazy during your detoxification. Even the most stubborn cravings and addictions will be curved. People who already detoxed claim the incredible change in as little as 24 hours and their desires have lessened

Grains and Gluten

Gluten is the two most common food sensitivities. Most people do not realize that they are sensitive to certain foods because this condition is not a real allergy like shellfish or peanut allergy, which creates hives, close the throat, swell the tongues, and can kill the person within minutes.

Unlike true allergies, food sensitivity is a subtle reaction to food. It is hidden because the small changes usually occur in the digestive tract. When you have food sensitivities, the lining in the gastrointestinal tract, particularly the intestine gradually becomes damaged and porous, a condition called a leaky gut, wherein food particles enter the bloodstream, creating a response to the body's immune system.

Earlier, I have mentioned about how the body protects itself and inflammation is a good sign that the body's defenses are working. However, when you have a leaky gut, your body is consistently in a state of low-grade inflammation as a reaction to the foreign particles in your bloodstream, resulting in many various symptoms that you would not connect to the food you eat. Some of these symptoms include brain fog, fatigue, depression, headaches, sinus problems, allergies, reflux, irritable bowel, autoimmune disease, joint pain, and skin diseases, such as eczema and acne.

Moreover, low-grade inflammation also triggers insulin resistance, which causes weight gain.

Gluten, a protein found in oats, spelled, rye, barley, and wheat. Some people are unable to digest it, causing a leaky gut. Additionally, because of genetic modification, a new strain of wheat has been created. This grain contains amylopectin A, a super-starch that triggers spikes in blood sugar. Two slices of bread made from this new corn raise the blood sugar more than 2 tablespoons of table sugar.

Gluten sensitivity, together with super-starch, triggers more inflammation, which increases the risk of diabetes and obesity.

All grains, including cereals, bread, and snacks, even the gluten-free kind, can spike blood sugar and insulin because they contain carbohydrates.

Moreover, research shows that when you eat high carb food, mainly if you have been consuming high-fructose food and your liver has been metabolizing fructose for quite some time, even when there is no fructose in your diet, your liver will convert the glucose, found in flour and bread, into fructose. Hence, during your detox, as mentioned earlier, you will need to avoid high carb food, such as rice, bread, and another non-vegetable carbohydrate.

Factory-Made and Processed Foods

As you already know, these foods are packed with artificial sweeteners and high-fructose corn syrup. They also made with preservatives, chemicals, additives, monosodium glutamate or MSG, and hydrogenated fats. MSG cause insulin spike, leading to cravings, hunger, and overeating.

During your detox, eat only food that is low-glycemic, contain good fats, proteins, phytonutrients, fiber, minerals, and vitamins.

Keep in mind; MSG can be hidden, so watch out for these ingredients:

- Any "flavoring" or "flavors."

- Anything with "enzyme modified."

- Anything with "hydrolyzed."

- Anything containing "enzymes."

- Anything with "glutamate" in it

- Autolyzed plant protein

- Autolyzed yeast

- Barley malt

- Bouillon and broth

- Carrageenan

- Gelatin

- Glutamate

- Glutamic acid

- Hydrolyzed plant protein (HPP)

- Hydrolyzed vegetable protein (HVP)

- Malt extract

- Maltodextrin

- Natural seasonings

- Protease

- Stock

- Textured protein

- Umami

- Vegetable protein extract

- Yeast extract

- Yeast food or nutrient

- Processed and Refined Vegetable Oils

You will need to avoid sunflower, canola, soybean oil, and more. They contain omega-6 fatty acids that cause inflammation. During your detox, use extra-virgin coconut butter or extra-virgin olive oil. Extra-virgin olive oil contains polyphenols, a potent antioxidant, and anti-inflammatory compounds while coconut butter contains anti-inflammatory fats, such as lauric acid, the same fat found in breast milk. If you need oil for high-heat cooking, grape seed oil is safe.

Alcohol

Alcohol is sugar in various forms. Moreover, when you drink alcohol, it impairs self-control, so you will be most likely to overeat mindlessly. It also contains 7 calories per gram, more than the four calories per gram of sugar. It not only causes leaky gut, but it also inflames the liver.

Caffeine

Some claim that caffeine speed up metabolism in a process called thermogenesis. However, you will also get the same effect by adding spices to your dishes, such as cayenne or jalapeno pepper. Caffeine is also addictive, and when inserted into sugary drinks, you will crave for more of that food. It also increases hunger. Like sugar, caffeine causes a surge of dopamine and then it wears off eventually. Even if you do not crave for coffee, you will undoubtedly desire for more sugar.

Avoiding caffeine will reboot your system, normalize brain chemistry and lessen cravings. Even decaf contain caffeine, so it is also off limits.

Starting Your Sugar Detoxification:

What Foods to Eat

When you've removed the bad stuff, now is the time to add the proper definite replacement. All the elements of your detox help your body detoxify, shed excess weight, and heal.

Avoiding the bad stuff and eating more of the excellent material optimize and accelerate your results.

Detox Pathway Boosters

To maximize your detox, you need to eat more superfoods and foods rich in phytonutrients. When your body is healthy, detoxification is smooth. When your body is toxic, especially when it's flooded with fructose, the liver gets sluggish, detox is slow, and certain toxins remain active longer than the system can handle. Hence, you get sick, and metabolism slows down. It also causes bloating, puffiness, and fluid retention.

When you are overweight, your body is high in toxins. As you lose weight during sugar detox, the toxins are released out from your fat tissues, and you will need to flush them out. Otherwise, it can impair weight loss and poison your metabolism.

Here are the foods the speed up detox:

- Watercress

- Wakame

- Rosemary

- Parsley

- Onion

- Lemon

- Kombu

- Kale

- Ginger

- Garlic

- Eggs

- Collards

- Cilantro

- Cayenne pepper

- Cauliflower

- Cabbage

- Brussels sprouts

- Broccoli

- Bok Choy

- Arame

They are rich in vitamin A and C, B vitamins, antioxidants, and phytonutrients.

Anti-Inflammatory Foods

Inflammation is your body's typical reaction to heal wounds and fight off bacteria. This is what happens when you have a sore throat, a cut, or strain. When the injury is infected, it turns, hot, red, and tender.

The inflammations that you need to be concerned about are the ones hidden inside your body and do not necessarily hurt. It's the inflammation caused by allergens, toxins, stress, bad food, the overgrowth of harmful bacteria in your gut, and low-grade infections.

Anything that causes inflammation will eventually cause insulin resistance, which produces belly fat and your body to hold on to fat cells. Earlier, I have mentioned the food that you need to avoid. Now I am going to give you the list of foods that will help minimize inflammation.

Omega 3 fatty acid-rich foods, such as:

- Salmon

- Eggs

- Grass-fed beef

- Hemp seeds

- Chia seeds

- Walnuts

- Flaxseeds

- Spices and herbs, such as turmeric

- Berries

- Dark-green leafy vegetables

- Extra-virgin olive oil

- Avocado

- Organic poultry

- Wild seafood

- Non-GMO tempeh and tofu

Foods That Cure Leaky Gut and Improve Gut Function

Every individual has 500 species of bacteria in the digestive system. These bacteria help control metabolism, digestion, and inflammation. Research studies also indicate that your weight may be controlled more by that the bacteria in your gut eat than what you eat yourself.

The bacteria in your gut increase, depending on what you eat and feed them. When you eat healthy food, the right bacteria grow and help boost your metabolism. However, if you eat junk, unhealthy diet, the harmful bacteria is the once that increase. This is something you should avoid because bad bacteria produce nasty gas and toxins that cause inflammation, weight gain, puffiness, bloated belly, and diabesity or the metabolic dysfunction. This is characterized by metabolic syndrome, insulin resistance, obesity, and type 2 diabetes, which is all caused by high blood sugar and can be treated using the same treatment.

When there is an imbalance of gut bacteria in your digestive system, it damages the lining of your gut or a leaky gut, which causes inflammation, and in turn, damages metabolism, affects how the brain controls appetite, leads to insulin resistance, and of course, weight gain.

Low sugar, low starch, high fiber, and whole food diet feeds the good bacteria and starves the harmful bacteria. Foods that are rich in minerals and vitamins help improve gut function. It includes:

- Bok Choy

- Pumpkin seeds

- Kale

- Arugula

- Carrots

- Tomatoes

- Turkey

- Salmon

- Chicken

- Parsley

- Onion

- Kimchi

These foods are high in vitamin A, zinc, antioxidants, amino acids, and probiotics.

Blood Sugar Balancers

The key to balance blood sugar is protein. Each meal should contain lean, preferably organic, animal protein, paired with delicious vegetables.

If you are a vegan or a vegetarian, you may have a serious weight and health problem when you substitute meat with starchy food, such as pasta, rice, bread, and other dense carbohydrate food, when once consumed turn into sugar and lead to cravings.

Even beans and grains can be a problem since these foods spike blood sugar and insulin more than animal protein. Eating all veggies can be unhealthy unless you know what you are doing.

Yes, you need to eat less factory-farmed meat, but animal-based protein is important for most people. If they come from pasture-raised or wild sources, then animal protein can be very healthy.

Your detox will partially depend on your current metabolism and health. The sicker you are, the less room you have regarding the sugar you can consume. As you detoxify and lose weight, your resilience will increase, and after the detox period, you can experiment with beans and grains as a source of protein. However, if you currently have significant health concerns, then avoid them, for the time being.

Seeds and nuts are the exceptions when it comes to protein from plant sources. They do not spike blood sugar and are great as snacks if you do not have nut allergies. They are particularly suitable for people with diabesity since they reduce the risk of diabetes, help with weight loss, and improve metabolism since they are packed with good fats, protein, minerals, such as zinc and magnesium, and fiber, all help reverse diabesity.

Exercise

Exercise is vital during your detox period. As little as 30 minutes of moderate exercise to begin your day will jump-start your metabolism and balance your hormones, blood sugar, and brain chemistry so that you can make better food choices during the day.

Exercise regulates appetite, reduces cravings, improves insulin sensitivity, and activates detox pathways to help eliminate toxins that cause weight gain, reduce inflammation, reduce stress hormone cortisol, and encourages better help.

Exercise is the best anxiety and depression treatment. It improves self-esteem, well-being, and energy.

If you already have an exercise routine, just continue to do whatever it is you enjoy for 30 minutes. If you haven't been exercising regularly, start with a 30-minute slow or brisk walking. If you can only do 5 minutes, then start with it and do it 2 times a day. Work your way up from there. Walking is the easiest and the most accessible exercise to everyone. It doesn't require any fancy equipment or memberships. You can also try out other physical activities.

Supplements

When it comes to health and weight loss, nutrients are vital. When the body is low in essential nutrients, it craves more food, seeking to get the nutrients it needs. Hence, you end up eating more, often sugary and junk foods, searching for the nutrients that are just not there. You overeat, but the body is still starving and not satisfied.

When you start to eat more real food, you will feel more satisfied, and you will eat less. However, your body will still need the essential amount of high-quality nutrients to help your body efficiently work. Sufficient amount of vitamins and minerals are required to burn calories, regulate appetite, boost detoxification, lower inflammation, regulate cortisol or stress hormones, aid digestion, and help the cells become more sensitive to insulin.

Hydrate

Most of us are frequently dehydrated. We become even more dehydrated because most of us love to drink caffeinated drinks. Staying hydrated is one of the keys to detoxification.

Fluid helps flush out environmental and metabolic toxins through the kidneys, increases energy, and improves regular bowel movements. Thus, drinking at least 8 glasses of water daily is essential during and after detox.

Studies reveal that we often mistake thirst for hunger, and eat instead of drinking. Always keep a bottle of fresh filtered water throughout the day and drink. Hydrate!

Write Your Experience

Keeping a journal and writing down your thoughts, feelings, and experiences unfiltered have been proven to reduce stress and help the process of detoxification. It's one of the best ways to stop the cycle of mindless eating. Journaling enables you to process your emotions and thoughts in a healthy, proactive way rather than just stuffing them down with bad habits and bad foods.

Writing will help you metabolize not just your thoughts, but also your calories better. Keeping an honest account of your experience is essential. Buy a blank notebook and write about your experience every morning and at night.

Unwind and Relax

Most of us are not motivated to take a break seriously. Consider this then: when the body is stressed, it causes a spike in insulin level, increase the level of cytokines or the immune system messenger molecules that cause inflammation, and increase the level of cortisol that causes accumulation of fat on the belly.

Stress also makes you hungrier and increases your cravings for sugar and carbohydrates, which trigger metabolic dysfunction, leading to excessive weight gain. So take time unwind and take a break. The breathing exercise below will help you relax.

5-Minute Relaxation Breathing

1. Sit down as comfortably as you can – on a chair, cross-legged on a cushion on the floor, or on a propped up pillows on your bed.

2. Close your mouth and eyes.

3. Breathe slowly through your nose, counting to 5 as you inhale.

4. Hold in 5 counts.

5. Slowly exhale, counting to 5 as you breathe out.

6. Repeat for 5 minutes.

Get Into the Rhythm

Whether we like it or not, our bodies evolved into biological organisms. Whether we listen to the signals that our body is sending us or not, it follows a specific rhythm – time to sleep, wake up, eat, relax, and exercise.

Simple behavioral changes will help you get back into the rhythm, which has powerful effects, including better sleep, increased energy, weight loss, and a lot more. Thus, during your detox period, create a schedule and stick to it.

Research shows that eating very late, skipping meals, and not eating breakfast screw up your metabolism. Not eating during the day results in the night-eating syndrome or binge eating at night or getting up in the middle of the night to feed. This causes diabesity, which results in blood sugar swings.

Wake up, sleep, eat, exercise, and relax the same time every day during your detox period. You will soon notice your body getting into the rhythm. The best thing about routines is that you won't have to waste mental energy continually planning your day. Eating an early breakfast will kick-start your metabolism and allow it to burn calories all day. Likewise, you need to avoid eating 2-3 hours before bedtime to prevent fat from being stored while you sleep. While you sleep, your body grows, rebuilds, and repairs itself. However, when you are sleeping, you are burning less energy, so the last thing you want is your belly growing.

Get Enough Sleep

Not getting sufficient sleep is linked to various diseases, including obesity. Since the invention of the light bulb, humans have been staying up longer and later because we can, which disrupts the body's sync with the natural rhythm of the seasons and mess up with the first sleep pattern.

If you don't get the right amount of sleep, it increases the production of ghrelin, the hunger hormone and it decreases the production of leptin, the appetite-suppressing hormone. When it comes to sugar, sleep is a natural appetite suppressant.

If you are working night shifts, you may have noticed that you are always craving for something sweet, like ice cream, cookies, and more. Your body is not getting enough energy because you are not getting enough sleep, so you eat to get the energy your body needs.

Now that you know what you need to avoid and what you need to get more of; let's get you ready to start your sugar detox.

Chapter 3: Preparing for Sugar Detox

The key to a successful sugar detoxification is a good plan and efficient preparation. Admit it; you probably spend more time planning vacations and parties than planning how to be healthy. Before you begin your detox, design your life for success and create an environment that will automatically direct you to make healthier choices. For instance, if you have nuts instead of donuts in your pantry, then you are more likely to make a healthy decision. Set your kitchen, your mind, and your school or work environment to maximize your detox. This is Day 1 and Day 2 – the unofficial start of your sugar detox.

Sugar Detox Your Kitchen

Your kitchen is probably packed with processed, sugar-packed, and junk food. You are going to start your detox with your kitchen. Throw away any items that fall under the following categories:

- Packaged, boxed, canned, or anything that is not real food. You can keep anything that is canned whole food, such as artichokes or sardines that contains a couple of real ingredients, such as salt or water.

- Drinks or foods that contain any form of sugar, including artificial sweeteners, organic cane juice, maple syrup, agave, molasses, and honey, mainly any fruit juices or beverages sweetened with sugar.

- Foods that contain refined vegetable oils, such as soybean or corn oil, and hydrogenated oil.

- Foods with dyes, coloring, additives, preservatives, or artificial sweeteners – anything that is processed in any way and has a label.

If you are unsure if the food or drink cuts, the best thing to do is get rid of it. Be thorough!

The following items also need to go. If you don't want to throw them, transfer them somewhere that is far from your eyesight during your detox. You need to avoid them while you are detoxifying. After your detox your body, you may introduce some them back into your diet.

- Products with gluten, including, pasta, bread, bagels, etc.

- All grains, including the ones that are gluten-free.

Supply Your Kitchen with the Good Stuff

Groceries

After clearing out your cabinets and fridge, it's time to fill them with real, whole, fresh food for your detox.

Make sure you have these staples.

- Almond meal

- Anti-inflammatory and Detoxifying herbs and spices, including turmeric, thyme, cayenne pepper, rosemary, cumin, chili powder, sage, onion powder, oregano, cinnamon, cilantro, coriander, parsley, and paprika

- Apple cider vinegar

- Balsamic vinegar

- Black pepper (peppercorns that you can freshly grind)

- Broth, low-sodium (chicken or vegetable)

- Coconut butter, extra-virgin, also known as coconut oil – it may be solid or liquid at room temperature

- Coconut milk, full-fat, canned

- Dijon mustard

- Jarred or canned Kalamata olives

- Nut butter (raw if possible; choose from almond, cashew, macadamia, or walnut)

- Nuts: almonds, walnuts, macadamia pecans,

- Olive oil, extra-virgin

- Other healthy oils that you like (walnut, sesame, grapeseed, flax, or avocado)

- Sea salt

- Seeds: chia, hemp, pumpkin, flax, sesame

- Tahini or sesame seed paste—great for salad dressings and in sauces for vegetables)

- Tamari, low-sodium, gluten-free

- Unsweetened almond or hemp milk

Depending on the meal plan or the dishes, you plan to prepare for the day or the week during your detox, add the specific ingredients needed; you may not need some of the ingredients listed above. Read on through the recipes, plan your meals, and then shop for the ingredients that you need.

You may think that buying fresh, whole, good food is expensive. However, if you consider how much money you spend on takeout food, convenience food, sodas, coffee, and junk food, you would be surprised that you are spending that much money on food that is toxic. You should also consider how much you would be paying treating diseases brought on by processed and poisonous foods. When you look at the long-term benefits on your health and wallet, choosing healthy foods is way better and healthier for you.

Detoxifying Bath Supplies

Relaxing at home is easy. Lavender oil, baking soda, and Epsom salt in your bath soak will not only help you relax; the combination creates a detoxifying and relaxing routine.

For each session, you will need the following:

- 2 cups Epsom salt

- 1/2 cup baking soda

- 10 drops lavender oil

Fill the tub with water as hot as you can handle. Add the Epsom salt, baking soda, and lavender oil. To make the bathroom more relaxing, you can play some soothing music and light candles. Soak in the tub for about 20-30 minutes.

This detoxifying bath will help you de-stress and relax for a better sleep. Your muscles and mind will benefit from this healing bath.

Sugar Detox Journal

Purchase a journal or notebook. Here you will record your experiences, thoughts, and results.

Supplements

Most people are deficient in necessary nutrients, especially people who haven't been taking care of their bodies. Before you start your detox, make sure you have the following on hand. They will supply your body with the essential nutrients that it needs. The combination is designed for long-term usage. You can find any of the supplements at your local health store.

Supplement	Dosage	Benefits
Alpha lipoic acid (ALA)	300-600 milligrams	Balances insulin and blood sugar; taken together with other supplements that optimize metabolism, blood sugar balance, and insulin.
Chromium	500-1000 micrograms	Balances insulin and blood sugar; taken together with other supplements that optimize metabolism, blood sugar balance, and insulin.
Cinnamon	500-1000 milligrams	Balances insulin and blood sugar; taken together with other supplements that optimize metabolism, blood sugar balance, and insulin.
Green tea catechins	100-200 milligrams	Balances insulin and blood sugar; taken together with other supplements that optimize metabolism, blood sugar balance, and insulin.

Magnesium citrate	200-300 milligrams (2-3 capsules) 1-2 times a day	This is used to manage constipation caused by PolyGlycopleX or PGX, mainly if your stomach is not used too much fiber. This also helps improve sleep, reduce anxiety, improve the control of blood sugar, and help cure muscle cramps.
Multivitamin and multimineral supplement	Take as indicated on the label	Help run the metabolism, improve insulin functioning, and balance blood sugar.

| PolyGlyco pleX or PGX (capsules or powder) | 2.5-5 grams before every meal; you can take additional doses during the day to control cravings | This super fiber slows down insulin and blood sugar spikes. It also reduces needs and makes you feel full longer. Take before every meal with a large-sized glass of water. The powder form works better than the capsule. This will also help you manage night eating or night cravings.

Drink the recommended eight glasses water daily to ensure the fiber moves through your body. |
|---|---|---|
| Purified fish oil (DHA/ EPA) | 2 grams | Balances blood sugar, sensitize insulin, anti-inflammatory, boosts brain function and prevents heart disease. |
| Vitamin D3 | 2,000 IU | |

Zinc	15-30 milligrams	Balances insulin and blood sugar; taken together with other supplements that optimize metabolism, blood sugar balance, and insulin.

Testing Tools to Monitor Your Progress

If you have the money or if your budget allows, you may want to get the following tools that will help you test and monitor your progress.

- A glucose monitor

- A weighing scale, preferably one who uploads your weight, body composition, and BMI; if possible, one that directly uploads your info to a smartphone.

- A blood pressure monitor, if possible, one that instantly uploads your info into a smartphone

- A personal movement track to track your daily sleep and activity

Exercise Clothing

The goal here is for maximum success. You will be more likely to exercise if you keep a pair of appropriate exercise clothing and your supplies in the same place. Whenever you are ready to go, you have everything you need. Get your sneakers out of the closet or buy a new pair. Choose to clothe that you are most comfortable with. Remove any obstacles so that when you start your detox, you are ready to go.

Water Filter and Bottle

The best way to drink pure, clean water is to filter your own using a simple carbon and then pour the water into a glass or stainless steel bottle. You can find these items in the supermarket or at the home-goods store.

Reduce Consumption of Sugar, Caffeine, and Alcohol

The 2-day preparation is the start of your detox, and during this period, you will start weaning yourself off from the sugar, alcohol, and caffeine. These substances will make you feel temporarily alert and energized, but their effects wear off fast and you'll end up in a vicious crash-and-crave cycle.

- It won't be easy getting off caffeine. Do it in stages. Reduce your usual amount to half during the first day, and then reduce again by half the second day. During the official first day of your detox, go cold turkey. Take a nap if you are tired. Lots of water, a gentle exercise, a hot bath, and 1, 000 mg twice daily of vitamin C can help reduce any a headache that you may experience because of withdrawal.

- Day 2 is the time to quit alcohol and any beverage that is sweetened with artificial sweeteners or sugar. This is also the time to stop eating processed food.

How Do I Deal with Detox Symptoms

During this phase, you have already started weaning yourself from sugar and processed foods so that you may feel hungry. You will also experience the typical signs of hunger, such as a vacant sensation in the chest or abdominal area and belly growling. You will crave for sweets and feel fatigued or light-headed between meals, have trouble completing a 30-minute walk, want for coffee, experience brain fog or have difficulty concentrating, and feel anxious, moody, or short-tempered.

Rest

Relax, nap, and rest. This is vital during the first few days of detox. Rest relaxes your nervous system, the system responsible for your fight or flight response during a stressful event, helps the body repair. The first 2 days of your detox are where detoxification magic happens. Your body will adjust, and you will feel less than great, so you need to rest. This will pass once your body has transitioned.

Accept the Detox Symptoms

Feeling not so great is a great sign. It means that your body is transitioning and eliminating the toxins from your body.

Flush the Toxins

Take a detoxifying bath, get a massage, enjoy a sauna, do stretching or a gentle yoga. All these things will help reduce inflammation and increase circulation in your body, which helps reduce soreness and achiness, increase chemical secretion, move toxins, and purify the body.

Get Things Moving

Clean bowels that efficiently working prevents constipation and headaches. Here are some tips to get things moving

- Drink lots of water to flush the kidneys and clean the intestines.

- Add 2 tablespoons ground flax seeds into your soups, salads, or shakes. These are rich in fiber and absorb plenty of water.

- Take 100-150 mg of magnesium citrate twice daily will help regular bowel movement. You can take as much as 6 capsules. Stop taking or reduce the amount if the bowel becomes too loose.

- Take 1000-2000 mg vitamin C one to two times

daily.

- Drink an herbal laxative, such as senna, cascara, or rhubarb before bedtime.

- Exercise helps things get moving. It's a powerful bowel stimulant and

- Sweat it out. Intense activity helps you sweat, which releases toxins through your skin. If your exercise does not cause you to sweat, take an infrared or steam sauna.

- Use an enema or suppository. There are available medications that you can buy at your local drugstore.

- Try liquid magnesium citrate. This is usually used to flush the bowel before a colonoscopy. If you can find this at your local drugstore, then you can use it. However, this solution is compelling. It can make you go in less than 4 hours, so don't leave the house and be ready.

- When all else fail, then it's time to see your doctor and find out what else is going on.

Move Your Body

A gentle exercise will help your circulation moving, flushing toxic fluid. Here's a simple yet effective way that can make a huge difference. Lie on your back close to a wall. Put your legs straight up against the wall and let it stay there for 20 minutes.

Take 2000 mg buffered vitamin C

One to two capsules daily will help relieve the detox symptoms.

Drink Lots of Fluids

Ensure that you are drinking a minimum of 8 glasses every day. You can also drink herbal teas if desired.

Eat!

Eat a lot when you are feeling it. Eat as much of the following non-starchy vegetables:

- Zucchini

- Watercress

- Turnip greens

- Tomatoes

- Swiss chard

- Summer squash

- Spinach

- Snow peas

- Snap beans

- Shallots

- Radishes

- Radicchio

- Parsley

- Palm hearts

- Onions

- Mustard greens

- Mushrooms

- Lettuces

- Kale

- Jalapeño peppers

- Green beans

- Gingerroot

- Garlic

- Fennel

- Endive

- Eggplant

- Dandelion greens

- Collard greens

- Chives

- Celery

- Cauliflower

- Cabbage

- Brussels sprouts

- Broccoli

- Bell peppers (red, green, yellow)

- Beet greens

- Bean sprouts

- Asparagus

- Arugula

- Artichoke

Don't Forget Your Snacks

To keep the hunger and craving away, include 2 snacks in your meal plan. A small protein-based dish with fiber and healthy fats, like sugar-free spreads or dips with veggies or nuts will help keep your energy up and your blood sugar steady. You can also cook your meals, adding a bit of extra to serve as your snack - snack doesn't necessarily mean nuts and spread. If you want, you can eat six small meals a day – some people find this easier.

Set Your Mind

You have to set your mind right. If you are thinking wrong and if you feel that you won't succeed, then you will head that way. It's not just healthy eating habits; it's also a positive mindset that will determine the success of your detox.

Your journal will help you root out your beliefs, attitudes, and mental obstacles that are preventing you from success. You need to be aware of the challenges so that you can shift your focus to what you want to achieve and how you can reach it.

During your 2-day preparation, focus on the questions below and write whatever comes to your mind. If other feelings and thoughts go to you when you are writing down your answers, then write them down as well. Writing down what happens to your mind makes you more accountable to yourself, and it can transform your inner desires into reality. Here are the questions that you need to answer.

- Why am I detoxifying? What can I achieve in my life

and my body with this detox?

- What three particular goals do I want to achieve during this detox?

- What are three particular things stopping me from achieving my weight goal? Is it sugar addiction? Emotional eating? Busy life? Always eating junk food? Fear of failure? Fear of success? Food pushers who advertise and encourage unhealthy food and eating habits?

- What beliefs hinder me from being healthy? Do I think I don't deserve much attention and time? Do I have this belief that being healthy is hard? I tried before, and it wasn't successful.

- Was it the way I overeat? Was it the way I eat food that is not nourishing?

- How do sickness and excess weight affect my ability to fulfill the things I want to do and make me happy?

- If I start eating healthy, how will my life change? If I take care of my health, how will it affect my life?

- How was my life when I was healthier and nurtured myself with care?

The more the obstacles and the benefits come into life, the better you will be able to get past them. More than that, the more connected you are to your intention and purpose, the more motivated you will be.

Be honest with yourself. Why are you detoxifying? Who are you doing this for? For yourself? For your loved ones? How different will your life be if you are healthy? The most important questions of all – will you be there to witness your children and grandchildren grow up? How long will you be able to spend time with your family and friends?

Measure Your Progress

The day before you start your detox, measure the following and record them in your detox journal.

Weight

Without clothes on, weigh yourself the very first thing in the morning when you wake up.

Height

Measure how tall you are in feet and inches.

Waist Size

Wrapping the tape measure around your belly button, measure the widest point of your waist, not the portion where your belt is located.

Hip Size

Same with the waist, measure the widest point around your hips.

Thigh Circumference

Same with the waist and hips, measure the widest point around each, individual thigh.

Blood Pressure

If you have a blood pressure cuff, then you can do this at home. If not, this can be done at the drugstore or by your doctor.

Now you are ready to start your sugar detox.

CHAPTER 4: WHAT TO EXPECT AND HOW TO GET THROUGH

You are officially starting your sugar detoxification – Day 3 to Day 14. It won't be an easy adjustment and transition. However, if you armed with the knowledge of what to expect and how to tips on how you can deal with the various symptoms, your journey will be more comfortable.

Day 3: This Is It!

This is the when most people usually experience flu-like symptoms, self-doubt, and low blood sugar. This is the start a very challenging journey. Hold on to your reigns! You are likely not experiencing real cold or flu, but you are experiencing the symptoms of sugar detox -this is a typical reaction, and it will subside after a couple of days.

Day 4: Ten More Days to Go!

You may notice your skin breaking out with pimples. This is

a normal and a great sign! Your detoxification is working, and your body is clearing out the toxins. You may also experience minor irritation on your skin and mood changes.

Day 5: I made it Through!

The cravings and the headaches will start to go away. If you are unprepared for hunger, slip-ups and temptations may happen. This is what your preparation is all about – having the right food and healthy snacks on hand, plus planning meals on time.

Day 6: Almost Half Way Done!

The flu or cold-like symptoms will begin to subside on this day. You can also check out your supply. The meal plans you have created, and the recipes to make sure you are still on point. It's also good to read the preparation tips once more.

Day 7: One Week Down!

This is where most people experience diarrhea, constipation, or bloating. Make sure you follow the tips given on how to avoid constipation.

Day 8: One More Week!

Over the weekend, you may feel the temptation and slip-off from your detox. If you haven't experienced fatigue early on, then this may be the day you will start to feel worn-out. You might start feeling tired of the food that you are eating and feel overwhelmed by how much preparation you need to do for your food.

If you slipped, don't be harsh on yourself. Instead, be more firm in your commitment. The recipes included in this book are also easy, and there are too many sugar-detox recipes online. Just make sure each recipe follows the guidelines mentioned above.

Day 9: Yeah! I Am Feeling Good! No More Cravings!

Gas, bloating, and other digestive issues will begin to clear. You may have collected a couple of recipes that you'd like to try and you are getting the hang of cooking. You can change and add any recipes you have clipped outside of this book into your meal plan.

You will also notice that you are no more extended craving more junk and sweet foods the way you did before you started detoxifying. Read your journal. Look back at your successes and your struggles. Your daily log will show you how far you have gone.

Day 10: I Feel A Bit Weak, But This Is Not As Hard As I Thought. I Should Continue Eating Healthy!

A low carb diet can result in weakness or shakiness. If you have been regularly working out, you will notice your performance is affected. Make sure you are getting enough healthy fat. This will be your primary source of energy since you have cut back on carbohydrates and sugar.

After the feeling of lethargy, you will feel the improvement in your energy and mood as you approach the end of your detox. You've now learned to surf on sugar-free waves.

Day 11: I Sleep Like a Baby, But I Am Craving For Something Sweet

By this day, you may notice that you are sleeping faster and better. You will also see that you feel refreshed and rested when you wake up in the morning. Ensure that you follow your waking and sleeping schedule.

However, you may feel the longing for the junk and sugary foods you usually eat, and you may get bored with the food choices. The excitement may pan out at eating healthy food. Again, search for more exciting sugar detox-friendly recipes. You can certainly add tons of recipes to your 2-week meal plan. You can even continue eating healthy for life!

Day 12: Am I Losing Any Weight? The Two Weeks Are Almost Up.

The sugar detox will help you shed the excess weight, but it won't help if you weigh yourself every day. It's ideal to consider yourself once before you start your detox and then after 14 days.

You may feel impatient with only two days to go! Your detox is almost over. Don't think about the detox. Instead, pamper and treat yourself. See a concert, go to a museum, get a manicure, and see a play. Anything that will distract you from what you are currently doing.

Day 13: Almost Done! What Do I Do After?

You may feel anxious that your detox will soon be over. You will now start planning to reintroduce some of the food that you have eliminated for this detox – beans, and dairy.

You may feel the urge to cheat since your detox is almost over. You may even call it enough since it's already day 13. Keep your goals in mind. This detox is not only about getting rid of sugar, but it's also about changing your unhealthy eating habits into a healthy one. When you make it through just one more day, the feeling of accomplishment will be awesome!

Day 14: I Made It!

Sheer joy! Excitement! Pride! Relief! You pushed through and made it! Tomorrow, you can start reintroducing back the food you were not allowed to eat during the past 2 weeks. Remember to add them back slowly to your diet.

Your Daily Ritual

Here's a reminder of what you need to do every day during your detox.

Morning

- At the start of your day, take your measurements. Write the result in your journal – glucose, blood pressure, etc. Also, take note how many hours of sleep you got and the quality of your sleep.

- Do your 30-minute exercise – brisk walking or your preferred exercise.

- Take your PGX fiber just before breakfast.

- If taking, take your supplement with your breakfast.

- Optional: Eat your choice of mid-morning snack.

Afternoon

- Take your PGX fiber just before lunch.

- Enjoy your lunch.

- Optional: Eat your choice of a mid-afternoon snack.

Evening

- Take your PGX fiber just before dinner.

- If taking, take your supplement.

- Enjoy your dinner

- Record your experience throughout the day. Jot down what you ate, what you did, how you felt, any changes and improvements in your focus and energy, and how these changes make you feel emotional, mentally, and physically. Write down any detox symptoms.

- Practice your choice of a 5-minute deep-breathing exercise.

- Sleep.

You are now ready to start your detox. Read on through the recipes and carefully plan your meal plan for two weeks. Choose from any of the following recipes or use whatever recipes are sugar detox-friendly.

Chapter 5: Sugar Detox Meal Plan Sample

A sugar detox diet is not as complicated as you think. Just make sure that you stay clear of the foods and products that you need to avoid during the period of your detoxification. Here's a sample of what your meals will look like. It's filled with super delicious real, whole foods that are good for you.

DAY 1	
Breakfast	Spinach and Cheese Baked Eggs
Mid-Morning Snack	Toasted Tamari-Rosemary Almond
Lunch	Sweet Pepper Cheesy Poppers
Mid-Afternoon Snack	3 pieces egg, hard-boiled, remove yolk if desired
Dinner	Baked Spinach-Stuffed Chicken
DAY 2	
Breakfast	Feta and Cucumber Relish

Mid-Morning Snack	Leftover Toasted Tamari-Rosemary Almond
Lunch	Leftover Baked Spinach-Stuffed Chicken
Mid-Afternoon Snack	Cheesy Spinach Dip
Dinner	Asian-Inspired Turkey Lettuce Cups
DAY 3	
Breakfast	Peanut Butter Smoothie
Mid-Morning Snack	3 pieces egg, hard-boiled, remove yolk if desired
Lunch	Leftover Asian-Inspired Turkey Lettuce Cups with Tossed mixed green salad with tomatoes, sweet peppers, cucumber, dressed with vinegar and extra-virgin olive oil
Mid-Afternoon Snack	Leftover Spinach and Cheese Baked Eggs
Dinner	Fresh Herb Marinated Grilled Chicken

DAY 4	
Breakfast	Mini Frittata's
Mid-Morning Snack	1 cheese stick
Lunch	Leftover Fresh Herb Marinated Grilled Chicken with Chicken and Cilantro Salad
Mid-Afternoon Snack	Celery dipped in sugar-free peanut butter or your preferred sugar-free nut butter
Dinner	Bean and Chicken Stew with Mini Cheesy Zucchini Bites
DAY 5	
Breakfast	Leftover Mini Frittata's
Mid-Morning Snack	Mediterranean-Inspired Spicy Feta Dip

Lunch	Leftover Bean and Chicken Stew with Tossed mixed green salad with tomatoes, sweet peppers, cucumber, dressed with vinegar and extra-virgin olive oil
Mid-Afternoon Snack	Tomato, Cucumber, and Feta Salad
Dinner	Cheesy Cauliflower Bread Sticks with Italian-Inspired Green Bean Salad
DAY 6	
Breakfast	Egg Muffin
Mid-Morning Snack	1/4 cup ricotta cheese (low fat, part-skim) tossed with a couple drops liquid vanilla stevia and 1/4 teaspoon vanilla extract
Lunch	Leftover Cheesy Cauliflower Bread Sticks with Italian-Inspired Green Bean Salad
Mid-Afternoon Snack	Mediterranean-Inspired Spicy Feta Dip
Dinner	Lemon-Garlic Chicken Drumsticks with Zucchini Salad
DAY 7	

Breakfast	Scrambled eggs with sautéed mushrooms and spinach with Homemade Salsa
Mid-Morning Snack	1/2 cup cottage cheese
Lunch	Vegetable Soup
Mid-Afternoon Snack	Leftover Toasted Tamari-Rosemary Almond
Dinner	Lemon-Garlic Chicken Drumsticks with Zucchini Salad

Optional After-Dinner Snacks:

- 1/4 cup ricotta cheese (low fat, part-skim) tossed with a couple drops liquid vanilla stevia and 1/4 teaspoon vanilla extract

- 1 cheese stick

- Vanilla-Flavored Chia Pudding

- Cucumber slices topped with cottage cheese (low-fat,

about ½ cup)

- 3 pieces egg, hard-boiled, remove yolk if desired

This simple sample meal plan is interchangeable, and you can adapt the recipes to your needs. If you want to customize your meal plan; feel free to search for sugar detox approved recipes and create your special one.

You may be doing this sugar detox solo and will have leftovers. You can scale down the ingredients to adjust the recipe for what you will need for the whole week.

Shopping List

Meats and Eggs	Dairy	Vegetables	Condiments or Miscellaneous
8 ounces pork sausage OR use ground turkey	8 ounces Gouda cheese, OR just use mozzarella	1 bag frozen green beans	1 jar sugar-free natural peanut butter
8 chicken drumsticks	2 packages (8-ounce each) cream cheese	1 bunch of fresh scallions or green onions	1 small-sized jar of sun-dried tomatoes
8 chicken breasts	2 cups Parmesan cheese	1 fresh head cauliflower	2 cans chicken broth, low-sodium

3 dozen eggs	2 cups feta cheese	1 pound fresh green beans	4 ounces chia seeds
1 pound ground turkey	1 package mozzarella cheese, shredded	1 pound mini sweet peppers	Fresh parsley, cilantro, and basil,
	1 package cheddar cheese, shredded	1 stalk celery	homemade hummus for snacking
	1 package cheese sticks	1-2 packages cherry tomatoes	homemade salsa
	1 container (16-ounce) cottage OR low-fat ricotta cheese	18 cups fresh spinach	homemade tomato sauce

	1 container (12-ounce) Greek yogurt, nonfat, plain	4-6 cucumbers	Low-sodium Tamari soy sauce
	1 carton unsweetened almond milk or your milk of choice	6-8 lemons	Powdered or liquid stevia extract
		8 fresh zucchini	Raw almonds
		8 sweet peppers, large-sized	Sesame seeds
		1 package (8 ounces) fresh mushrooms	Vinegar and olive oil to dress salad, also your choice of seasonings

		Frozen spinach	
		Garlic	
		Lettuce leaves for salad and Asian-Inspired Turkey Lettuce Cups	
		Onions, 2 white, and 1 red	

You can follow this meal plan or create your own. You may even know some recipes that are sugar detox-friendly. Feel free to use them.

CHAPTER 6: SUGAR DETOX RECIPES

Spinach and Cheese Baked Eggs

Serves: 6

Prep: 5 minutes

Cook: 15 minutes

Ingredients:

- 6 eggs

- 4 teaspoons olive oil, divided into 2 portions

- 2 teaspoons garlic, minced, divided into 2 portions

- 12 cups fresh spinach, divided into 2 portions

- 1 cup cheese, shredded, divided into 2 portions (I used mozzarella, low-fat)

Directions:

1. Preheat the oven to 350F.

2. Pour 2 teaspoons olive oil into a large-sized skillet.

3. Add 1 teaspoon garlic and 1/2 of the spinach. Sauté for about 2 to 3 minutes or until wilted. Add 1/2 of the cheese and then stir to combine 2 well.

4. Grease 3 ramekins with nonstick cooking spray. Divide the spinach mixture between the ramekins.

5. Cook the remaining ingredients as directed above and then divide between 3 more greased ramekins.

6. Carefully crack 1 egg over each spinach mixture.

7. Bake in the preheated oven for about 15 minutes for slightly runny yolks or bake until the desired doneness.

8. Season each serving with pepper and salt. Top with some fruit. Serve!

Toasted Tamari Almond Snack

Serves: 4

Prep: 5 minutes

Cook: 5 minutes

Ingredients:

- 2 tablespoons tamari soy sauce

- 1 cup almonds, raw

- 1 tablespoon fresh rosemary, chopped, optional

Directions:

1. Toast the raw almonds in a dry sauté pan over medium heat. Toss and cook until the almonds begin to smell delicious.

2. Remove the pan from the heat.

3. Carefully add 1 tablespoon tamari and, if using, rosemary, into the pan. Return to the burner and cook, continually stirring, until the sauce is absorbed and there are no more juices left.

4. Let slightly chill before serving.

5. Store in an airtight container for up to 7 days.

Sweet Pepper Cheesy Poppers

Serves: 30

Prep: 15

Cook: 15

Ingredients:

- 1 pound mini sweet peppers, halved

- 1/2 cup feta cheese, crumbled

- 1/4 cup onion, grated

- 2 cloves garlic, minced

- 2 tablespoons cilantro, chopped

- 8 ounces cream cheese, at room temperature

- 8 ounces smoked Gouda cheese, grated

Directions:

1. Preheat the oven to425F.

2. Except for the peppers, put all of the ingredients into

99

a bowl and mix until combined.

3. Fill each sweet pepper half with the cheese mixture.

4. Bake in the preheated oven for 15 to 18 minutes or until the cheese is melty and slight browned.

Baked Stuffed Chicken &Spinach Recipe

Serves: 10

Prep: 10 minutes

Cook: 30 minutes

Ingredients:

- 1 cup frozen spinach, heated, excess water drained

- 1 cup marinara sauce, preferably homemade

- 1 cup ricotta cheese, part-skim

- 1 egg, beaten

- 1/2 cup mozzarella cheese, shredded

- 1/2 teaspoon salt

- 10 pieces (4 ounces) chicken breast, thin, OR 5 pieces (8-ounce) breasts, sliced into halves

- Pepper, to taste

Directions:

1. Preheat the oven to 375F.

2. Put the spinach, ricotta, egg, pepper, and salt into a mixing bowl and combine.

3. Grease a 9x13-inch baking dish with nonstick cooking spray.

4. Put the chicken breast into the greased dish. Evenly divide the spinach mixture between the chicken and put the portions on top of each breast. Roll the chicken and arrange them in the bowl with the seam side facing down.

5. Pour the marinara sauce evenly over the chicken breasts. Sprinkle all over with the mozzarella cheese.

6. Bake in the preheated oven for about 35 to 40 minutes or until the sauce is bubbling and the cheese is melted.

Feta and Cucumber Relish

Serves: 4

Prep: 10 min

Cook: 0 min

Ingredients:

- 1 cup cucumber, peeled and then chopped

- 1 cup fresh tomato, chopped

- 1 scallion, chopped

- 1 tablespoon extra-virgin olive oil

- 1/2 cup feta cheese, crumbled

- Salt and pepper, to taste

Directions:

1. Put all of the ingredients into a bowl and mix until combined.

2. Serve immediately. If not, refrigerate until ready to serve.

Feta and Sun-Dried Tomato Frittata

Serves: 4

Prep: 5 minutes

Cook: 10 minutes

Ingredients:

- 1 clove garlic, minced

- 1/2 cup egg whites

- 1/2 cup light feta cheese, crumbled

- 1/2 cup onion, diced

- 1/2 cup sun-dried tomato, drained, chopped

- 1/4 cup almond milk, unsweetened

- 2 eggs

- 2 scallions, chopped

- 2 teaspoons coconut oil or olive oil

Directions:

1. Put the oil in a medium-sized oven-safe skillet and heat. When the oil is hot, add the onion and garlic. Sauté until the onion is translucent.

2. Add the tomatoes. Cook for about 2 to3 minutes or until heated through.

3. Meanwhile, crack the eggs, milk, and egg whites into a small-sized bowl and whisk to combine.

4. Pour the egg mixture into the skillet. Evenly sprinkle the feta cheese over the top of the egg mixture.

5. Reduce the heat to low and cook the egg mixture until the middle is almost set and the edges are set.

6. Transfer the skillet to the oven and broil for about 3 to 5 minutes or until the middle is no longer runny.

7. If desired, top with additional feta cheese and scallions.

Spinach Cheesy

Serves: 7

Prep: 5 minutes

Cook: 5 minutes

Ingredients:

- 4 ounces Neufchatel cheese, OR lite cream cheese

- 4 cups spinach, packed into the measuring cup

- 2 teaspoons olive oil

- 1/4 teaspoon salt

- 1/4 cup Parmesan cheese

- 1 cup ricotta cheese, part-skim

- 1 clove garlic, chopped

Directions:

1. Put the oil in a sauté pan and heat. Add the garlic and spinach, Sprinkle with salt and sauté until wilted. Set aside to cool

2. Put the Neufchatel and ricotta cheese into a blender. Blend until the mixture is smooth.

3. Add the Parmesan and cooled spinach. Pulse for 5 to 7 times or until the ingredients are incorporated – DO NOT OVER BLEND.

4. Serve immediately or refrigerate until ready to serve. Serve with your fresh raw veggies kabob– cherry tomatoes, broccoli, peppers, and cucumbers.

Asian Turkey Lettuce Cups

Serves: 4

Prep: 15 minutes

Cook: 20 minutes

Ingredients:

- 1 carrot, large, shredded

- 1 pound ground turkey

- 1 red or yellow bell pepper, large-sized, diced

- 1 tablespoon fresh ginger, minced

- 1/2 cup mushrooms, sliced

- 1/2 cup water

- 1/2 teaspoon salt

- 1/2 teaspoon sesame seeds

- 1/4 cup fresh herbs, chopped: basil, cilantro, or mint

- 1/4 teaspoon Emeril's Asian Essence powder

- 1/4 teaspoon garlic powder

- 1/4 teaspoon ground cinnamon

- 2 tablespoons homemade hoisin sauce

- 2 teaspoons coconut oil or olive oil

- 4 Bibb or Boston lettuce leaves, large-sized

Directions:

1. Put the oil into a large skillet and heat. Add the ginger and the turkey. Cook until the turkey is browned.

2. Add the mushrooms, pepper, hoisin sauce, and water into the skillet. Cook until heated through. Add the Asian essence, cinnamon, garlic powder, and salt. Let heat for 1 minute.

3. Wash the lettuce leaves and dry. Add 1 1/2 cups of the turkey mixture into each lettuce leaf.

4. Sprinkle the turkey mixture with the carrots, herbs, and sesame seeds.

Peanut Butter Smoothie

Serves: 1

Prep: 2 minutes

Cook: 0 minutes

Ingredients:

- 1/2 cup cottage cheese, low fat

- 1/2 cup almond milk, unsweetened

- 1 tablespoon peanut butter, natural, no sugar added

- 1 scoop Whey protein, optional

- 2 full droppers liquid stevia (plain, vanilla, or toffee flavor)

- 1 cup ice

Optional toppings:

- Cacao Nibs

- Peanut butter, to drizzle

Directions:

1. Put all the ingredients in a blender. Blend until the mixture is smooth.

Fresh Herb Marinated Grilled Chicken

Serves: 4

Prep: 10 minutes

Cook: 30 minutes

Ingredients:

- 1 cup mixture of fresh herbs, leaves only, loosely packed (parsley, basil, cilantro)

- 1/4 cup lemon juice

- 1/4 cup olive oil

- 1/4 teaspoon pepper

- 2 large garlic cloves

- 3 pieces (about 1 pound) chicken breasts, boneless, skinless, rinsed, patted dry, sliced lengthwise into halves

- 3 teaspoons salt

Directions:

2. Wash the herbs and then chop them. Put into a high-powered blender or food processor. Add the lemon juice, oil, pepper, salt, and garlic; process until smooth.

3. Put the chicken into a Ziploc bag. Add the marinade, seal the bag, and massage to coat the meat with the marinade. Put the container in the fridge and let marinate for at least 30 minutes and up to 8 hours.

4. When ready to serve, grill the chicken breasts for about 10-15 minutes per side or until cooked through – the meat no longer meat and the juices run clear.

Vegetable Soup

Serves: 8

Prep: 10 minutes

Cook: 40 minutes

Ingredients:

- 1 cup carrots, sliced

- 1 cup green beans, frozen

- 1 cup onion, chopped

- 1/2 teaspoon garlic powder

- 1/2 teaspoon salt

- 1/4 teaspoon pepper

- 2 cloves garlic, large-sized, minced

- 2 cups celery, sliced

- 2 cups fresh spinach, chopped

- 2 cups vegetable stock or chicken broth, low sodium

- 2 teaspoons olive oil

- 4 cups water

Optional:

- 1 cup cannellini beans,

- 1 cup shelled edamame or soybeans

- 1/2 cup fresh parsley, chopped,

- Parmesan cheese, grated

Directions:

1. Put the oil into a Dutch oven and heat over medium heat. Add the garlic and sauté until fragrant.

2. Add the celery, onion, and carrots. Sauté for about 10 minutes or until the veggies are tender.

3. Pour the broth and the water into the Dutch oven and bring to a boil.

4. When boiling, add the green beans and, if using, the soybeans. Add the seasonings.

5. Cover the pot and reduce the heat to low. Simmer for 30 minutes.

6. Remove the cover. Add the parsley and spinach. Cook for about 5 minutes or until the spinach is wilted.

Vanilla-Flavored Chia Pudding

Serves: 2

Prep: 5 minutes

Cook: 0 minutes

Ingredients:

- 1/3 cup chia seeds

- 1 teaspoon vanilla extract

- 1 teaspoon liquid stevia, vanilla flavored

- 1 cup almond milk, unsweetened

- Whipped Cream, dairy-free, optional

Directions:

1. Put all the ingredients in a large pitcher and whisk until combined.

2. Divide between 2 serving glasses.

3. Refrigerate for about 10 minutes or until set.

4. If desired, top each serving with whipped cream.

Notes: You can adjust the amount of liquid stevia. Start with 1/4 teaspoon and increase the amount to taste.

Mini Frittatas

Serves: 12

Prep: 10 minutes

Cook: 30 minutes

Ingredients:

- 8 ounces pork sausage

- 2 egg whites

- 2 cups yellow and red sweet peppers, diced

- 10 eggs

- 1/4 teaspoon pepper

- 1/2 teaspoon salt

- 1/2 cup pepper jack cheese

- 1/2 cup 1% milk

Optional:

- Fresh Cilantro, Chopped

- Green Onions

- Salsa, homemade

- Sour Cream, homemade

Directions:

1. Preheat the oven to 350F.

2. Cook the sausage in a skillet over medium heat until cooked through.

3. With a slotted spoon, transfer the cooked sausage to a plate and set aside.

4. In the same skillet, add the peppers and sauté until soft.

5. Crack the eggs into a large-sized bowl. Add the milk and egg whites. Whisk until combined.

6. Divide the peppers and sausage into 12 muffin cups. Pour the egg mixture into each muffin cup. Sprinkle 1 heaping tablespoon cheese over each.

7. With a fork, stir the contents of the muffin cups to

combine.

8. Bake in the preheated oven for about 25 to 30 minutes.

Chicken and Cilantro Salad

Serves: 4

Prep: 10 minutes

Cook:

Ingredients:

- 6 ounces chicken breast, cooked and chopped

- 4 yellow or red peppers, tops cut off and the insides scooped out, OR large-sized tomatoes, cut into halves, and the insides scooped out

- 1/2 cup red onion, diced

- 1/2 cup cherry tomatoes, halved

- 1 cup celery, diced

For the dressing:

- 2 tablespoons fresh cilantro, chopped

- 1/2 teaspoon salt

- 1/2 teaspoon cumin

- 1/2 cup Greek yogurt, nonfat, plain

- 1 teaspoon lemon juice

- 1 teaspoon garlic powder

- 1 tablespoon extra-virgin olive oil

Directions:

1. Put all of the dressing ingredients into a small-sized bowl and mix until combined.

2. Except for the peppers or tomatoes, put the rest of the ingredients into a large sized bowl. Add the dressing and toss to coat.

3. Put about 1 cup of the chicken salad into each tomato half or pepper.

Bean and Chicken Stew

Serves: 12

Prep: 10 minutes

Cook: 3 hours

Ingredients:

- 2 cups chicken, cooked, shredded

- 4 cups chicken broth, low-sodium

- 3 teaspoons garlic, minced

- 1/2 teaspoon salt

- 2 teaspoons cumin

- 1/2 teaspoon oregano

- 1 can hominy or corn, drained and then rinsed

- 1 can black beans, drained and then rinsed

- 1 cup salsa, homemade, OR 1 can diced tomatoes

- 1 can Lima/butter beans, Or cannellini beans,

drained and rinsed

- 1/2 cup sour cream, homemade

Optional toppings:

- Fresh cilantro

- Cheese, shredded

- Chives

- Sour cream

Directions:

1. Except for the sour cream and the optional toppings, put all of the ingredients into a crockpot. Mix to combine. Cover and cook for 3 hours on HIGH.

2. When the cooking time is up, add the sour cream to the pot and mix until well incorporated.

3. Cover the pot and cook on LOW for 30 minutes.

4. Serve topped with your preferred toppings

Mini Cheesy Zucchini Bites

Serves: 3

Prep: 5 minutes

Cook: 15 minutes

Ingredients:

- 1 egg

- 1/2 cup Parmesan cheese, grated

- 1/4 cup fresh cilantro, chopped, optional

- 2 cups zucchini, grated (about 2 to 3 medium-sized)

- Salt and pepper, to taste

Directions:

1. Preheat the oven to 400F.

2. Grease a mini muffin pan with nonstick cooking spray.

3. Put the zucchini, cheese, egg, and cilantro in a bowl. Mix until combined.

4. Evenly divide the zucchini mixture between the mini muffin cups. Fill each cup to the top, patting them down if needed to pack the cups.

5. Bake for about 15 to 18 minutes or until the edges are golden brown. Check after 15 minutes.

Mediterranean-Inspired Spicy Feta Dip

Serves: 8

Prep: 10 minutes

Cook: 0 minutes

Ingredients:

- 1 cup feta cheese, reduced fat, crumbled

- 1 lemon, juice only

- 1/4 cup almond milk, unsweetened

- 1/4 cup chopped walnuts, toasted

- 1/4 cup Greek yogurt, nonfat, plain

- 1/4 cup red peppers, roasted, chopped

- 1/4 teaspoon pepper

- 1/4 teaspoon Tabasco sauce, homemade

- 2 teaspoons extra-virgin olive oil

- Kalamata or green olives, optional, for topping

Vegetables to dip:

- Celery

- Seedless cucumbers

- Carrots

Directions:

1. Put all of the ingredients into a blender or a food processor. Pulse or blend until the mixture reaches your desired consistency.

2. Transfer to a serving bowl. If desired, top with more olives and red peppers.

3. Serve immediately or keep refrigerated until ready to serve.

Cheesy Cauliflower Bread Sticks

Serves: 4

Prep: 5 minutes

Cook: 40 minutes

Ingredients:

- 1 cup mozzarella cheese, shredded

- 1 cup Parmesan cheese, grated

- 1 teaspoon garlic powder

- 1 teaspoon Italian seasonings

- 1/2 teaspoon salt

- 2 egg whites, OR 1/4 cup egg whites

- 4 cups cauliflower, chopped (about 1 head cauliflower, washed clean and dried)

- Marinara sauce, homemade

Directions:

1. Preheat the oven to 450F.

2. Line 2 pieces of 8x12-inch baking sheets with parchment paper.

3. Microwave the cauliflower for about 7 to 8 minutes or steam for about 20 minutes or until tender.

4. Put the cooked cauliflower into a food processor; pulse until resembling rice.

5. Transfer the cauliflower rice to a large-sized bowl. Add the Parmesan cheese, seasonings, and egg whites. Mix until well combined.

6. Spread the cauliflower mixture into an even layer in one of the prepared baking sheets.

7. Put the baking sheets into the oven and bake for about 30 minutes or until the tops are browned.

8. Invert the cauliflower into the other prepared baking sheet. Put in the oven and Bake for about 10 minutes or until the tops are browned.

9. Sprinkle the top with mozzarella cheese. Broil for

about 1 minute or until the cheese is melted.

10. Let rest for 10 minutes and then slice into 24 portions.

Italian-Inspired Green Bean Salad

Serves: 10

Prep: 5 minutes

Cook: 5 minutes

Ingredients:

- 1 1/2 pounds fresh Italian green beans, OR any kind

- 1 cup cherry tomatoes, halved

- 1/2 cup fresh basil, chopped

- 1/2 cup red onion, sliced

- 1/4 cup fresh flat or curly leaf parsley, chopped

- 2 cups English cucumber, sliced with the skin on

- 2 ounces Pecorino Romano cheese, chunks

For the Italian dressing:

- 1 lemon, juice and zest

- 1/2 teaspoon garlic powder

- 1/2 teaspoon salt

- 1/4 teaspoon pepper

- 2 tablespoons extra-virgin olive oil

- 2 tablespoons red-wine vinegar

Directions:

1. Bring a large-sized pot with water to a boil. When the water is boiling, add the beans. Blanch for 5 minutes. Immediately drain and then put the beans into an ice bath – a bowl filled with ice and water. Let fresh for about 5 to 10 minutes.

2. When the beans are chilled, drain and put into a serving bowl. Add the remaining ingredients to the pan.

3. Put all of the Italian dressing ingredients into a small-sized bowl and whisk until combined. Pour the dressing over the salad ingredients.

4. Gently toss to coat. If needed, adjust pepper and salt to taste.

5. Serve immediately or refrigerate until ready to serve.

Egg Muffin

Serves: 1

Prep: 2 minutes

Cook: 2 minutes

Ingredients:

- 1 tablespoon cheese, shredded, your choice

- 1 tablespoon cream, OR milk

- 1/2 scallion, chopped

- 3 egg whites, OR 1 egg

- Nonstick cooking spray

- Salt and pepper to taste

Directions:

1. Grease a small-sized dish or a custard ramekin with nonstick cooking spray.

2. Put the egg whites/egg and cream into the dish. Whisk to combine.

3. Add the scallion and cheese. Loosely cover the dish with a paper towel and put the plate in the microwave; microwave for about 50 to 60 seconds. If your microwave had a scrambled eggs setting, use that. Do not microwave for too long or you will have a significant mess.

Lemon-Garlic Chicken Drumsticks

Serves: 8

Prep: 5 minutes

Cook: 20 minutes

Ingredients:

- 8 chicken drumsticks

- 3 cloves garlic, minced

- 2 tablespoons olive oil

- 2 lemons, juice only

- 1/4 cup fresh parsley, chopped

- 1/2 tablespoon butter

- 1 teaspoon salt

- 1 teaspoon pepper

- 1 teaspoon dried Italian Seasonings

- 1 lemon, zest only

Directions:

1. Put the olive oil in a large-sized sauté pan and heat.

2. While the pan is heating, season the chicken drumsticks with pepper, salt, and Italian seasoning.

3. When the oil is hot, put the chicken into the pan and cook until all the sides are browned. Transfer the drumsticks to a plate and cover with foil to keep warm.

4. Reduce the heat to low. In the same skillet, add the butter and garlic, stir for about 1 to 2 minutes. Add the lemon zest and juice. Return the drumsticks to the pan.

5. Cover and let simmer for 20 minutes.

6. Coat the drumsticks with the sauce and transfer the drumsticks to a serving plate. Pour the remaining sauce over the chicken. Garnish with chopped fresh parsley. Serve!

Zucchini Salad

Serves: 6

Prep: 10 minutes

Cook: 0 minutes

Ingredients:

- 4 zucchini, medium-sized, shredded (about 6 cups)

- 1 lemon, zest only

- 1/2 teaspoon salt

- 1/4 cup fresh parsley and basil, chopped

- 2 lemons, juice only, OR 3 tablespoons lemon juice

- 3 tablespoons extra-virgin olive oil

- Pepper, to taste

Optional toppings:

- Dried cherries

- Goat cheese

- Almonds, sliced

Directions:

1. Slice, dice, or shred the zucchini to get 6 cups total. Put into a large-sized bowl.

2. Put the oil, lemon zest and juice, pepper, and salt into a small-sized bowl and whisk until combined.

3. Pour the dressing over the zucchini. Add the parsley and basil. Gently toss to coat.

4. If desired, top with extra toppings.

5. Serve immediately or keep refrigerated until serving time.

Homemade Salsa

Serves: 11

Prep: 5 minutes

Cook: 5 minutes

Ingredients:

- 1 can (28 ounces) whole peeled tomatoes, drained

- 1 cup onion, chopped

- 1 cup red pepper, chopped

- 1 tablespoon olive oil

- 1 whole jalapeno pepper, seeds and membrane removed, chopped

- 1 whole lime, juice only

- 1/2 cup fresh cilantro, chopped

- 1/2 teaspoon ground cumin

- 1/2 teaspoon salt

- 2 cans (10 ounces each) diced tomatoes with chilies

- 2 cloves garlic, chopped

Directions:

1. Put all of the ingredients into a food processor. Pulse 5 times for a chunky salsa or vibration up to 10 times for restaurant style.

2. Keep refrigerated.

FINAL WORDS

Thank you again for purchasing this book!

I really hope this book is able to help you.

The next step is for you to **join our email newsletter** to receive updates on any upcoming new book releases or promotions. You can sign-up for free, and as a bonus, you will receive a free gift. Our *"Health & Fitness Mistakes You Don't Know You're Making"* book! This book has been written to demystify, expose the top do's and don'ts and to finally equip you with the information you need to get in the best shape of your life. Due to the overwhelming amount of mis-information and lies told by magazines and self-proclaimed "gurus", it's becoming harder and harder to get reliable information to get in shape. As opposed to having to go through dozens of biased, unreliable and un-trustworthy sources to get your health & fitness information. Everything you need to help you has been broken down in this book for you to easily follow and to immediately get results to achieve your desired fitness goals in the shortest amount of time.

Once again, to join our free email newsletter and to receive a free copy of this valuable book, please visit the link and signup now:

www.hmwpublishing.com/gift

Finally, if you enjoyed this book, then I would like to ask you for a favor, would you be kind enough to leave a review for this book? It would be greatly appreciated!

Thank you and good luck in your journey!

ABOUT THE CO-AUTHOR

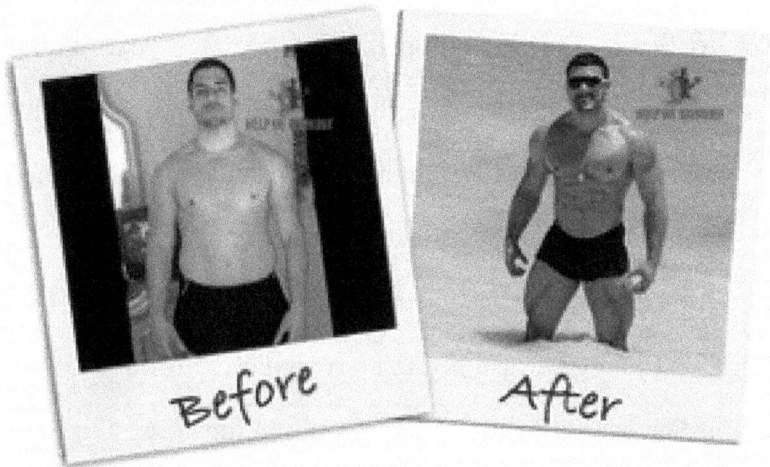

Before / After

My name is George Kaplo; I'm a certified personal trainer from Montreal, Canada. I'll start off by saying I'm not the biggest guy you will ever meet and this has never really been my goal. In fact, I started working out to overcome my biggest insecurity when I was younger, which was my self-confidence. This was due to my height measuring only 5 foot 5 inches (168cm), it pushed me down to attempt anything I ever wanted to achieve in life. You may be going through some challenges right now, or you may simply want to get fit, and I can certainly relate.

For me personally, I was always kind of interested in the health & fitness world and wanted to gain some muscle due to the numerous bullying in my teenage years about my height and my overweight body. I figured I couldn't do anything about my height, but I sure can do something about how my body looked like. This was the beginning of my transformation journey. I had no idea where to start, but I just got started. I felt worried and afraid at times that other people would make fun of me for doing the exercises the wrong way. I always wished I had a friend that was next to me who was knowledgeable enough to help me get started and "show me the ropes."

After a lot of work, studying and countless trial and errors. Some people began to notice how I was getting more fit and how I was starting to form a keen interest in the topic. This led many friends and new faces to come to me and ask me for fitness advice. At first, it seemed odd when people asked me to help them get in shape. But what kept me going is when they started to see changes in their own body and told me it's the first time that they saw real results!

From there, more people kept coming to me, and it made me realize after so much reading and studying in this field that it did help me but it also allowed me to help others. I'm now a fully certified personal trainer and have trained numerous clients to date who have achieved amazing results.

Today, my brother Alex Kaplo (also a Certified Personal Trainer) and I own & operate this publishing venture, where we bring passionate and expert authors to write about health and fitness topics. We also run an online fitness website "HelpMeWorkout.com" and I would love to connect with by inviting you to visit the website on the following page and signing up to our e-mail newsletter (you will even get a free book). Last but not least, if you are in the position I was once in and you want some guidance, don't hesitate and ask... I'll be there to help you out!

Your friend and coach,

George Kaplo
Certified Personal Trainer

Download another book for Free

I want to thank you for purchasing this book and offer you another book (just as long and valuable as this book), "Health & Fitness Mistakes You Don't Know You're Making", completely free.

Visit the link below to signup and receive it:

www.hmwpublishing.com/gift

In this book, I will break down the most common health & fitness mistakes, you are probably committing right now, and I will reveal how you can easily get in the best shape of your life!

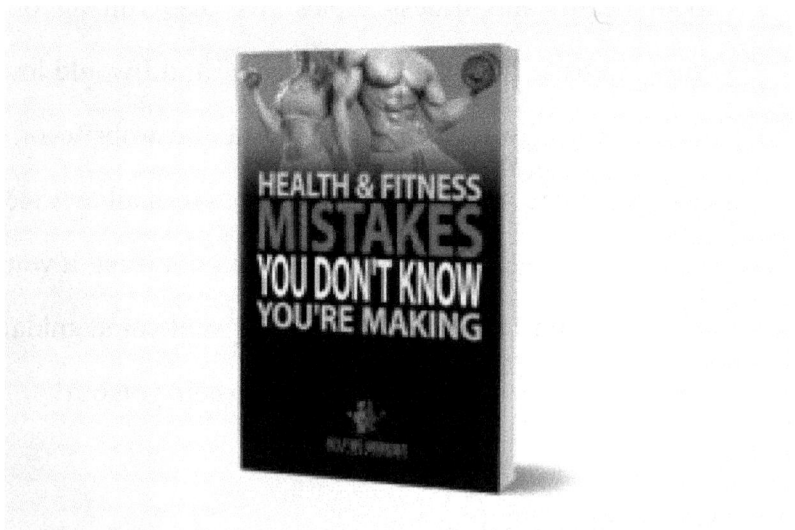

In addition to this valuable gift, you will also have an opportunity to get our new books for free, enter giveaways, and receive other valuable emails from me. Again, visit the link to sign up:

www.hmwpublishing.com/gift

HMW Publishing

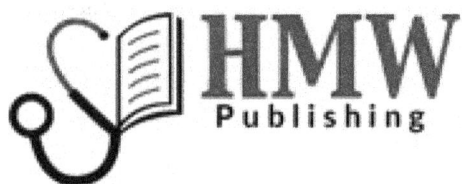

For more great books visit:

HMWPublishing.com

www.ingramcontent.com/pod-product-compliance
Lightning Source LLC
Chambersburg PA
CBHW050729030426
42336CB00012B/1482